Building a Sustainable Workout Routine:

A Comprehensive Guide for Beginners to Achieve Effective Exercise" (Health-care Tips)

Matthew R.Passmore

Table of Content

Chapter 1

Introduction

In a world where the pace of life often feels relentless and demanding, the pursuit of a healthy and balanced lifestyle has never been more crucial. Regular exercise is a cornerstone of this quest, offering a multitude of benefits for the body and mind. However, starting and maintaining a workout routine can be a daunting challenge, especially for beginners.

This comprehensive guide is designed to be your steadfast companion on the journey to building a sustainable workout routine. Whether you're a complete novice in the world of fitness or someone who has struggled to stick to an exercise plan, this book is here to provide you with the knowledge, guidance, and motivation you need to succeed.

We'll embark on a holistic exploration of exercise, delving into not only the physical aspects of working out but also the mental and emotional facets. You'll learn how to set achievable goals, select the right exercises for your needs, structure a balanced workout plan, and, most importantly, make exercise an integral and enjoyable part of your life.

As we progress through the chapters, you'll discover the art of warming up and cooling down, the significance of proper nutrition and hydration, and the secrets of effective rest and recovery. We'll also delve into the psychology of motivation, helping you stay on track, overcome obstacles, and celebrate your accomplishments.

Moreover, this guide recognizes the importance of sustainability not only in your health but in the broader context of the world we inhabit. We'll explore environmentally friendly workout practices and mindful approaches to exercise, fostering a deep commitment to both personal well-being and the planet's health.

So, if you're ready to embark on a transformative journey toward a healthier, more vibrant you, let's turn the page and begin your adventure. Building a sustainable workout routine is not just about enhancing your physical strength; it's about empowering yourself to lead a more fulfilling life.

1.1 Understanding the Importance of Exercise

Exercise, often regarded as a chore or a task, is far more than just a means to an end. It's a fundamental component of a healthy and fulfilling life. In this chapter, we'll delve into the myriad reasons why exercise matters, going beyond the aesthetics and exploring its profound impact on your physical, mental, and emotional well-being.

Physical Benefits:

Enhanced Fitness: Regular exercise improves cardiovascular health, boosts endurance, and increases strength. It's not just about looking good; it's about feeling strong and capable.

Weight Management: Exercise is a key player in maintaining a healthy weight. It helps burn calories, build muscle, and regulate your metabolism.

Disease Prevention: A consistent exercise routine can reduce the risk of chronic diseases, such as heart disease, diabetes, and certain types of cancer.

Improved Immune Function: Exercise can bolster your immune system, making you more resilient to infections and illnesses.

Better Bone Health: Weight-bearing exercises promote bone density, reducing the risk of osteoporosis and fractures.

Mental and Emotional Benefits:

Stress Reduction: Physical activity triggers the release of endorphins, which are natural mood lifters. It's a powerful stress-buster.

Mental Clarity: Exercise has been shown to enhance cognitive function, sharpening your focus and memory.

Better Sleep: Regular physical activity can lead to improved sleep quality, helping you wake up refreshed and energized.

Mood Regulation: Exercise is a potent tool for managing and preventing depression and anxiety. It can be a natural antidepressant.

Emotional Well-Being:

Boosted Self-Esteem: Achieving fitness goals and taking care of your body can boost your self-confidence and self-esteem.

Increased Energy: Contrary to what some might think, exercise provides you with more energy to tackle daily tasks and challenges.

Social Connection: Group activities and team sports provide opportunities for social interaction and building strong, supportive relationships.

As you begin your journey towards a sustainable workout routine, keep these benefits in mind. They are the reasons why you're committing to this path, and they will serve as a source of inspiration on days when motivation wanes. Understanding the importance of exercise is the first step toward transforming your life for the better.

1.2 Setting Goals for a Sustainable Workout Routine

Setting well-defined and achievable goals is the compass that will guide you on your journey towards a sustainable workout routine. Without clear objectives, it's easy to lose motivation and direction. In this chapter, we'll explore the art of goal setting and how it can drive your fitness endeavors.

Why Set Goals?

Goals serve as your exercise roadmap, giving purpose and structure to your workouts. Here are some compelling reasons to set specific fitness goals:

Motivation: Having a clear goal to work towards provides the motivation to stay committed to your workout routine, especially during challenging times.

Progress Tracking: Goals allow you to measure your progress. By regularly assessing your achievements, you can stay on course and make adjustments as needed.

Focus: Goals help you concentrate your efforts on what matters most to you. They prevent distractions and keep you on track.

Sense of Achievement: Achieving your fitness goals provides a sense of accomplishment and boosts your self-esteem.

Types of Goals:

Outcome Goals: These are overarching objectives, such as losing a certain amount of weight or running a specific distance within a set time frame. Outcome goals give you a big-picture view of what you want to achieve.

Behavioral Goals: These are the daily or weekly actions you take to reach your outcome goals. They focus on the behaviors needed to make progress, like working out a certain number of days each week or consuming a balanced diet.

Short-Term and Long-Term Goals: Short-term goals help you make progress quickly and maintain motivation. Long-term goals set the ultimate destination for your fitness journey. It's crucial to balance both types for sustained success.

SMART Goals:

One effective approach to goal setting is using the SMART criteria:

Specific: Define your goals with precision. Avoid vague objectives like "getting in shape." Instead, specify "losing 10 pounds" or "running a 5K race."

Measurable: Ensure your goals are quantifiable. You should be able to track your progress and know when you've achieved them.

Achievable: Set realistic goals that you can reasonably attain. Unrealistic objectives can lead to frustration and demotivation.

Relevant: Your goals should align with your broader values and aspirations. They should be personally meaningful.

Time-Bound: Set a timeframe for your goals. This creates a sense of urgency and helps you maintain focus.

Goal-Setting Strategies:

Start Small: Begin with achievable goals that build your confidence. As you achieve these, you can gradually increase the challenge.

Write Them Down: Document your goals and revisit them regularly. This reinforces your commitment.

Share Your Goals: Telling friends or family about your fitness goals can provide accountability and support.

Stay Flexible: Be open to adjusting your goals as needed. Life can be unpredictable, and flexibility can help you stay on track.

Remember that setting goals is not about perfection but progress. Your goals are unique to your aspirations and current fitness level. They will evolve as you do. Setting and working towards these goals will keep you motivated and help you build a sustainable workout routine

Chapter 2

Getting Started

Starting a workout routine, especially as a beginner, can be both exciting and daunting. In this chapter, we'll explore the essential steps to help you embark on your fitness journey with confidence.

1. Assessing Your Current Fitness Level:

Before you jump into a workout routine, it's crucial to assess your current fitness level. This evaluation serves as your starting point and helps you avoid overexertion or unrealistic expectations. Here are some ways to assess your fitness:

Physical Examination: Consider your overall health, any existing medical conditions, and your readiness for exercise. If you have concerns, consult a healthcare professional.

Fitness Tests: You can perform basic fitness tests like measuring your heart rate, assessing flexibility, and estimating your endurance and strength. These tests provide insights into your starting point.

Self-Assessment: Reflect on your daily activity level and lifestyle. Are you sedentary, moderately active, or already somewhat active? Understanding your habits is a key part of your assessment.

2. Choosing the Right Types of Exercises:

Once you have a clear understanding of your fitness level, it's time to select the right types of exercises that suit your goals and preferences. Here are some considerations:

Aerobic Exercises: These include activities like walking, jogging, cycling, and swimming. They are excellent for cardiovascular health and weight management.

Strength Training: This involves exercises with weights or resistance bands to build muscle and increase metabolism.

Flexibility and Balance Training: Activities such as yoga and Pilates can improve flexibility, balance, and posture.

Sports and Recreational Activities: Engaging in sports or recreational activities you enjoy can make exercise more fun and sustainable.

3. Start Gradually:

One common mistake beginners make is trying to do too much, too soon. It's important to ease into your workout routine to prevent injury and burnout. Consider these tips:

Set Realistic Goals: Begin with achievable targets. It could be as simple as walking for 20 minutes a day.

Progressive Overload: Gradually increase the intensity, duration, or frequency of your exercises. This allows your body to adapt and improve over time.

Listen to Your Body: Pay attention to any discomfort or pain. Soreness is common, but pain should not be ignored.

4. Get the Right Gear:

Depending on your chosen activities, you may need appropriate workout gear. This can include comfortable clothing, supportive footwear, and, for some activities, specific equipment.

5. Create a Comfortable Workout Space:

If you're working out at home, make sure you have a space that's conducive to exercise. Clear out clutter, ensure good ventilation, and have any necessary equipment ready.

Starting your fitness journey as a beginner is an important step towards a healthier and more active lifestyle. By assessing your fitness level, choosing the right exercises, and beginning gradually, you'll set a strong foundation for a sustainable workout routine. Remember, consistency and patience are key to long-term success

2.1 Assessing Your Current Fitness Level

Before diving into a new exercise routine, it's crucial to assess your current fitness level. This self-evaluation not only helps you understand where you stand in terms of physical fitness but also ensures your safety and sets the stage for setting realistic goals. Here's how to effectively assess your current fitness level:

1. Consult with a Healthcare Professional:

If you have any existing medical conditions or concerns about your health, it's wise to consult with a healthcare professional, such as your primary care physician. They can provide valuable insights into your physical condition and offer guidance on what types of exercises may be safe and beneficial for you

2. Self-Reflection:

Take some time to reflect on your current lifestyle and physical activity levels. Ask yourself questions like:

How active am I in my daily life? Am I mostly sedentary, moderately active, or already somewhat active?
Are there any physical limitations or injuries that I need to be aware of?

What are my fitness goals, and what specific areas do I want to improve (e.g., cardiovascular endurance, strength, flexibility)?

3. Basic Fitness Assessments:

Performing simple fitness assessments can provide valuable data about your current physical condition. These assessments can include:

Heart Rate: Measure your resting heart rate in the morning before getting out of bed. A lower resting heart rate typically indicates better cardiovascular fitness.

Flexibility: Assess your flexibility by attempting basic stretches and observing your range of motion in various joints.

Endurance: Time yourself walking or jogging a specific distance (e.g., 1 mile) or measure how long you can sustain physical activity without fatigue.

Strength: Determine your baseline strength by attempting bodyweight exercises like push-ups, squats, or planks.

4. Body Composition:

Understanding your body composition, including your body mass index (BMI) and body fat percentage, can provide insights into your overall health. This information can be obtained using various methods, including body composition scales or measurements taken by a fitness professional.

5. Record Your Baseline Measurements:

Once you've gathered the data from your assessments, record it for reference. This baseline information will serve as a starting point for tracking your progress as you continue with your exercise routine.

6. Be Realistic:

It's important to be honest and realistic about your current fitness level. This assessment is not about judgment but rather about understanding where you are and where you want to go. It's a critical step in setting achievable fitness goals.

Remember that everyone's starting point is different, and that's perfectly okay. What's most important is your commitment to improving your fitness and overall well-being. With a clear understanding of your current fitness level, you can create a workout plan that is tailored to your needs, ensuring a safe and effective journey towards your fitness goals

2.2 Choosing the Right Types of Exercises

Selecting the right types of exercises is a pivotal decision in crafting an effective and sustainable workout routine. The choice of exercises should align with your fitness goals, preferences, and individual needs. Here's how to make informed decisions:

1. Clarify Your Fitness Goals:

Begin by defining your fitness goals. What are you looking to achieve with your workout routine? Common goals include:

Weight loss or maintenance
Cardiovascular fitness and endurance
Strength and muscle development
Improved flexibility and balance
Stress reduction and mental well-being
Understanding your goals will guide your exercise choices, ensuring that they are purposeful and tailored to your objectives.

2. Variety is Key:

A well-rounded exercise routine often includes a mix of different types of exercisesThis diversity not only keeps your workouts interesting but also ensures that you target various aspects of fitness. The main categories of exercises to consider include:

Aerobic or Cardiovascular Exercises: These activities, such as walking, jogging, cycling, swimming, and dancing, elevate your heart rate and enhance cardiovascular fitness. They are excellent for weight management and overall health.

Strength Training Exercises: Strength exercises, using weights, resistance bands, or bodyweight, help build muscle, increase metabolism, and enhance functional strength. Squats, push-ups, and weightlifting are examples.

Flexibility and Balance Training: Activities like yoga, Pilates, and stretching routines improve flexibility, balance, and posture. They can also reduce the risk of injury.

Sports and Recreational Activities: Engaging in sports or recreational activities you enjoy, such as tennis, basketball, or hiking, can make exercise more fun and keep you motivated.

3. Consider Your Preferences:

Exercise should be enjoyable to ensure long-term commitment. Think about the types of activities you enjoy. If you love being outdoors, consider outdoor exercises like hiking or biking. If you prefer group settings, explore fitness classes or team sports. The more you enjoy your chosen activities, the more likely you are to stick with your routine.

4. Adapt to Your Fitness Level:

As a beginner, it's important to start with exercises that match your current fitness level. Gradually increase the intensity and complexity of your workouts as you gain experience and confidence. This prevents injury and ensures a sustainable progression.

5. Seek Professional Guidance:

If you're unsure about which exercises are suitable for you, consider consulting a fitness professional or personal trainer. They can create a tailored workout plan that aligns with your goals and helps you avoid common pitfalls.

6. Be Mindful of Safety:

Always prioritize safety in your exercise choices. Pay attention to proper form and technique to minimize the risk of injury. If you have any pre-existing health conditions or concerns, consult with a healthcare provider to ensure that your chosen exercises are safe for you.

By considering your goals, preferences, fitness level, and safety, you can choose the right types of exercises that set you up for a successful and sustainable workout routine. Remember that exercise should enhance your life, and the journey can be as rewarding as the destination.

Chapter 3

Creating a Workout Plan

Creating a structured workout plan is essential for building a sustainable and effective exercise routine. A well-designed plan not only keeps you on track but also ensures you target all the key areas of fitness. In this chapter, we'll guide you through the process of crafting a workout plan that suits your needs.

1. Set Clear and Specific Goals:

Your workout plan should align with your fitness goals. These goals should be clear, specific, and measurable. For example, if your goal is to improve cardiovascular fitness, you might aim to jog for 30 minutes without stopping within three months.

2. Determine the Frequency of Exercise:

How often you work out is a fundamental decision. Aim for a balanced approach. Most experts recommend at least 150 minutes of moderate-intensity aerobic activity or 75 minutes of vigorous-intensity aerobic activity per week. This can be broken down into sessions lasting 20-30 minutes. Strength training should be incorporated at least two days a week.

3. Choose the Right Exercises:

Select exercises that align with your goals. For example, if you're focusing on strength, include exercises like squats, push-ups, and weightlifting. For improved flexibility, add yoga or Pilates to your plan.

4. Structuring Your Weekly Workout Schedule:

Here's a sample weekly workout schedule:

Day 1: Cardiovascular Workout (e.g., 30 minutes of brisk walking or cycling)

Day 2: Strength Training (focus on different muscle groups, e.g., upper body)

Day 3: Rest or Gentle Activity (like yoga)

Day 4: Cardiovascular Workout (e.g., 20 minutes of jogging)

Day 5: Strength Training (focus on different muscle groups, e.g., lower body)

Day 6: Rest or Gentle Activity (like stretching)

Day 7: Cardiovascular Workout (e.g., swimming or dancing)

This is just an example. You can tailor your weekly schedule to suit your preferences and availability. The key is to include a variety of exercises while allowing for rest and recovery.

5. Progression and Variation:

To keep your workouts effective and engaging, consider the principles of progression and variation. Increase the intensity, duration, or complexity of your exercises gradually. This prevents plateaus and maintains motivation.

6. Warm-up and Cool Down:

Always incorporate a warm-up and cool-down into your workout plan. These are essential for injury prevention and recovery. A warm-up might include light cardio and dynamic stretches, while a cool-down could involve static stretching and deep breathing.

7. Track Your Progress:

Regularly track your progress to stay motivated and ensure you're on the right path to achieving your goals. Keep a workout journal or use fitness apps to record your sessions, and periodically reevaluate your goals.

8. Adapt to Your Lifestyle:

Your workout plan should be adaptable to your lifestyle. If you have a busy schedule, look for ways to incorporate shorter, high-intensity workouts. The key is to find a routine that you can sustain over the long term.

Creating a workout plan is a dynamic process. It may require adjustments as you progress and your goals change. The most important factor is consistency. Stick to your plan, stay motivated, and enjoy the benefits of a healthier, more active lifestyle

3.1 Structuring Your Weekly Workout Schedule

A well-structured weekly workout schedule is the cornerstone of a successful and sustainable exercise routine. It provides a framework for achieving your fitness goals while ensuring variety and balance in your workouts. Here's how to create an effective weekly workout schedule:

1. Define Your Goals:

Begin by clarifying your fitness goals. Knowing what you want to achieve will help shape your workout schedule. Whether it's weight loss, strength gain, improved cardiovascular health, or overall fitness, your goals will guide your choices.

2. Determine the Number of Weekly Workouts:

The frequency of your workouts should align with your goals and your fitness level. A general guideline for aerobic exercise is at least 150 minutes of moderate-intensity exercise or 75 minutes of vigorous-intensity exercise per week, accompanied by strength training on at least two days.

3. Mix Different Types of Workouts:

A balanced weekly schedule includes various types of workouts to address different aspects of fitness:

Cardiovascular Workouts: These include activities like running, cycling, or swimming to boost your heart rate and endurance. Aim for three to four sessions per week, each lasting 20-45 minutes.

Strength Training: Incorporate strength training exercises on two to three non-consecutive days per week. Target different muscle groups in each session.

Flexibility and Mobility: Include stretching, yoga, or Pilates to improve flexibility and mobility. Aim for 2-3 sessions per week.

4. Create a Weekly Workout Calendar:

Map out your workouts on a calendar. Here's an example of a balanced weekly workout schedule:

Monday: Cardiovascular Workout (e.g., running or brisk walking for 30 minutes)

Tuesday: Strength Training (focus on upper body)

Wednesday: Flexibility and Mobility (yoga or stretching)

Thursday: Cardiovascular Workout (e.g., cycling for 45 minutes)

Friday: Strength Training (focus on lower body)

Saturday: Rest or Active Recovery (gentle activities like swimming or a nature walk)

Sunday: Flexibility and Mobility (yoga or stretching)
5. Warm-Up and Cool Down:

Don't forget to include warm-up and cool-down periods in every workout. A warm-up should last 5-10 minutes and could include light cardio and dynamic stretching. The cool-down should last 5-10 minutes and consist of static stretching and deep breathing to help your body recover.

6. Progression and Adaptation:

As you progress, gradually increase the intensity, duration, or weight in your workouts. Periodically reassess your goals and make adjustments to your schedule as needed.

7. Rest and Recovery:

Rest days are essential to allow your body to recover and prevent overtraining. Listen to your body, and if you're feeling overly fatigued or experience pain, take the necessary rest.

8. Stay Flexible:

Life can be unpredictable, and your schedule should allow for flexibility. If you miss a workout or need to reschedule, don't be discouraged. Simply adapt and continue with your plan.

A well-structured weekly workout schedule provides the foundation for achieving your fitness goals while maintaining a sustainable and enjoyable exercise routine. Consistency is key, and with the right plan in place, you're on your way to a healthier and more active lifestyle

3.2 Incorporating Cardio, Strength, and Flexibility Exercises

Incorporating a balance of cardiovascular (cardio), strength, and flexibility exercises into your fitness routine is essential for overall well-being. Here's how to effectively integrate these three components into your workout plan:

1. Cardiovascular (Cardio) Exercises:

Cardio exercises are essential for heart health and improving endurance. Here's how to incorporate cardio into your routine:

Choose Activities You Enjoy: Select cardio activities that you find enjoyable, such as jogging, cycling, swimming, dancing, or group fitness classes. Enjoying the activity will make it easier to stick with it.

Set Goals: Define specific cardio goals, such as running for a certain distance, swimming for a set time, or walking a certain number of steps daily.

Schedule Regular Cardio Sessions: Aim for at least 150 minutes of moderate-intensity aerobic exercise or 75 minutes of vigorous-intensity aerobic exercise per week. Break this down into manageable sessions, such as 30 minutes, five times a week, or shorter, more frequent sessions.

2. Strength Training Exercises:

Strength training helps build muscle, boost metabolism, and enhance functional strength. Here's how to incorporate strength training into your routine:

Choose the Right Exercises: Focus on compound movements that engage multiple muscle groups. Examples include squats, deadlifts, bench presses, and bodyweight exercises like push-ups.

Frequency: Aim for strength training sessions on at least two non-consecutive days each week. This allows your muscles to recover between sessions.

Progressive Overload: Gradually increase the weight or resistance you use to challenge your muscles and stimulate growth. This can involve adding more weight to your dumbbell exercises or increasing the intensity of bodyweight exercises.

3. Flexibility and Mobility Exercises:

Flexibility and mobility exercises are often neglected but are crucial for injury prevention and joint health. Here's how to incorporate flexibility and mobility exercises into your routine:

Dedicated Sessions: Plan dedicated flexibility and mobility sessions into your weekly schedule. Yoga and Pilates are excellent choices for improving flexibility and mobility.

Warm-Up and Cool-Down: Include stretching and mobility exercises in your warm-up and cool-down routines for all your workouts. This helps improve your range of motion and prevents injury.

Proper Technique: Focus on proper stretching techniques, such as dynamic stretching before your workout and static stretching after. Breathe deeply and hold stretches for 15-30 seconds.

4. Create a Balanced Weekly Schedule:

To ensure a balanced fitness routine, create a weekly schedule that incorporates all three components. Here's a sample weekly schedule:

Day 1: Cardiovascular Workout (e.g., running or cycling)

Day 2: Strength Training (upper body focus)

Day 3: Flexibility and Mobility (yoga or stretching)

Day 4: Cardiovascular Workout (e.g., swimming or brisk walking)

Day 5: Strength Training (lower body focus)

Day 6: Active Recovery (gentle activities or a nature walk)

Day 7: Flexibility and Mobility (Pilates or stretching)

Adjust this schedule to fit your goals and preferences while ensuring a balanced mix of cardio, strength, and flexibility exercises.

By incorporating these three components into your fitness routine, you'll experience a comprehensive and well-rounded approach to fitness that supports your overall health, strength, and flexibility

Chapter 4

Proper Warm-up and Cool Down

A proper warm-up and cool-down are crucial components of any effective exercise routine. They help prepare your body for physical activity and aid in recovery after workouts. Here's how to incorporate these essential steps into your fitness plan:

Warm-Up:

A warm-up is a series of gentle exercises and movements that gradually raise your heart rate, increase blood flow to your muscles, and prepare your body for more intense activity. The primary goals of a warm-up are to prevent injury, enhance performance, and mentally prepare for your workout.

1. Cardiovascular Component:Incorporate light aerobic activity into your warm-up, such as brisk walking, slow jogging, or cycling at a low intensity. This helps increase your heart rate and circulation.

2. Dynamic Stretches:

Include dynamic stretches to mobilize your joints and muscles. These stretches involve controlled movements that take your joints and muscles through their full range of motion. Examples include leg swings, arm circles, or hip rotations.

3. Activation Exercises:

Perform exercises that activate the specific muscle groups you'll be using during your workout. For instance, if you're doing a strength training session that focuses on your legs, do bodyweight squats or leg lifts to engage those muscles.

4. Gradual Progression:

Your warm-up should gradually increase in intensity but remain low to moderate in effort. Start slowly and build up the intensity over 5-10 minutes.

Cool-Down:

The cool-down phase helps your body recover and gradually return to its resting state after exercise. It's an important part of reducing muscle soreness and preventing injury.

1. Low-Intensity Cardio:

After your main workout, engage in low-intensity aerobic activity like walking or slow cycling. This helps your heart rate gradually return to its normal range.

2. Static Stretches:

Perform static stretches, holding each stretch for 15-30 seconds. Focus on the major muscle groups you've worked during your workout. Examples include hamstring stretches, quad stretches, and shoulder stretches.

3. Deep Breathing:

Incorporate deep breathing exercises to relax and reduce tension. Take slow, deep breaths and focus on calming your body and mind.

4. Hydration and Nutrition:

Rehydrate by drinking water after your workout. Consume a balanced meal or snack within a couple of hours to replenish energy and support muscle recovery.

5. Reflect and Record:

Use the cool-down time to reflect on your workout and your progress. Consider keeping a workout journal to record your achievements and set new goals for future sessions.

Incorporating proper warm-up and cool-down routines into your exercise plan helps reduce the risk of injury, improve performance, and support your body's recovery. These steps are essential for a safe and effective fitness regimen, whether you're engaging in cardio, strength training, or flexibility exercises

4.1 Importance and Techniques for Warming Up

Warming up is a crucial step in any exercise routine, whether you're about to engage in cardiovascular activities, strength training, or flexibility exercises. It prepares your body physically and mentally for the main workout and offers several important benefits:

1. Injury Prevention:

Warming up gradually increases your heart rate and circulation, which in turn raises the temperature of your muscles. This increased muscle temperature enhances their elasticity and reduces the risk of strains and tears during exercise.

2. Improved Muscle Performance:

As your body temperature rises, your muscle fibers become more flexible and efficient. This enables better muscle contractions, leading to improved performance and strength during your workout.

3. Enhanced Range of Motion:

A proper warm-up helps increase joint lubrication and flexibility. This makes it easier to move through a full range of motion, reducing the risk of joint injuries and improving overall exercise quality.

4. Mental Preparation:

Warming up provides a mental transition from the activities of daily life to the focused state needed for exercise. It can help you get into the right mindset, increasing your workout's effectiveness.

Now, let's explore techniques for a proper warm-up:

1. Cardiovascular Component:

Start your warm-up with light aerobic activity to gradually increase your heart rate and circulation. This can include brisk walking, slow jogging, stationary cycling, or jumping jacks. The goal is to get your heart rate up but not to the level of your main workout.

2. Dynamic Stretches:

Incorporate dynamic stretches to mobilize your muscles and joints. These stretches involve controlled movements that take your joints and muscles through their full range of motion. Examples include leg swings, arm circles, and hip rotations. These movements help improve flexibility and blood flow to the muscles.

3. Activation Exercises:

Include exercises that activate the specific muscle groups you'll be using during your main workout. For example, if you're planning a strength training session that focuses on your legs, perform bodyweight squats or leg lifts. Engaging these muscles helps prepare them for more intense exercise.

4. Gradual Progression:

Your warm-up should gradually increase in intensity and duration, lasting 5-10 minutes. Start slowly and build up to a moderate level of effort. The goal is to prepare your body, not exhaust it.

Remember that the specific warm-up techniques can vary depending on the type of exercise you'll be doing. A warm-up for running may differ from one for weightlifting or yoga. Tailor your warm-up to the activity you're about to engage in to maximize its benefits and ensure a safe and effective workout

4.2 Cooling Down to Prevent Injuries and Enhance Flexibility

The cooling down phase of your workout is a crucial but often overlooked component of a well-rounded exercise routine. Cooling down involves performing specific exercises and stretches after your main workout to help your body transition from a state of intense physical activityto a state of rest. It serves several important purposes, including injury prevention and the enhancement of flexibility. Here's why and how to cool down effectively:

Importance of Cooling Down:

Injury Prevention: After a workout, your muscles and joints are warm and flexible. Abruptly stopping intense exercise can lead to muscle cramps, strains, and even injuries. A proper cool-down allows your body to gradually return to its resting state, reducing the risk of injury.

Reduced Muscle Soreness: Cooling down aids in the removal of metabolic waste products, such as lactic acid, which accumulate during exercise. Clearing these byproducts from your muscles more efficiently can help reduce muscle soreness and stiffness.

Enhanced Flexibility: The post-workout period is an opportune time to work on flexibility. Your muscles are warmed up and more receptive to stretching. Regularly incorporating stretching exercises during your cool-down can lead to improved flexibility over time.

Techniques for Cooling Down:

Low-Intensity Cardio: After your primary workout, engage in low-intensity aerobic activity such as brisk walking, light jogging, or gentle cycling. This gradually lowers your heart rate and allows your cardiovascular system to return to its resting state.

Static Stretches: Incorporate static stretches into your cool-down routine. These stretches involve holding a position for 15-30 seconds without bouncing. Focus on stretching major muscle groups you've worked during your workout, such as hamstrings, quadriceps, calves, and shoulders. This can help improve flexibility.

Deep Breathing: Use deep breathing exercises to relax and reduce post-workout tension. Take slow, deep breaths and concentrate on calming both your body and mind. Deep breathing can be especially effective for reducing stress and anxiety that might have built up during the workout.

Hydration and Nutrition: After your workout, ensure that you rehydrate by drinking water, especially if you've perspired heavily. It's also important to consume a balanced meal or snack within a couple of hours to replenish energy and support muscle recovery.

Reflection and Planning: Use the cool-down period to reflect on your workout. Consider what went well, what could be improved, and any changes you want to make in your routine. If you keep a workout journal, this is an ideal time to record your achievements and set new goals.

A proper cool-down doesn't need to be time-consuming. Spending 5-10 minutes on these cooling down techniques is often sufficient. By incorporating a thorough cool-down into your workout routine, you can reduce the risk of injuries, support muscle recovery, and enhance your flexibility over time. This contributes to a safer, more effective, and enjoyable fitness journey

Chapter 5

Nutrition and Hydration

Proper nutrition and hydration are essential components of a successful workout routine. What you eat and drink can significantly impact your energy levels, exercise performance, recovery, and overall health. Here's how to optimize your nutrition and hydration for effective workouts:

1. Pre-Workout Nutrition:

Before your workout, it's important to fuel your body with the right nutrients for optimal performance. Here are some pre-workout nutrition tips:

Carbohydrates: Complex carbohydrates, like whole grains, fruits, and vegetables, provide a steady source of energy. Consuming them 1-2 hours before your workout can help fuel your muscles.

Protein: Protein is crucial for muscle repair and growth. Include a small amount of lean protein in your pre-workout snack to support muscle health.

Hydration: Start your workout well-hydrated. Drink water throughout the day and consider consuming a small amount of water or a sports drink 15-30 minutes before exercising toprevent dehydration.

2. During Exercise Hydration:

Proper hydration during exercise is vital to maintain energy, prevent overheating, and ensure your body functions optimally. Here are some guidelines for staying hydrated during your workout:

Water: For most moderate-intensity workouts, water is sufficient for staying hydrated. Take small sips regularly during your exercise session.

Electrolytes: If you're engaged in prolonged, intense exercise or sweating heavily, consider a sports drink to replenish lost electrolytes like sodium and potassium.

3. Post-Workout Nutrition:

After your workout, your body requires nutrients for recovery and muscle repair. Consider these post-workout nutrition recommendations:

Protein: Consume a source of protein within 30 minutes to two hours after exercise to support muscle recovery. Options include lean meats, poultry, fish, eggs, or plant-based protein sources like tofu or legumes.

Carbohydrates: Replenish glycogen stores by consuming carbohydrates, especially if your workout was intense and prolonged. Whole grains, fruits, and vegetables are excellent choices.

Hydration: Rehydrate by drinking water after your workout to replace any fluids lost during exercise. You can also consume a sports drink if your workout was particularly strenuous and you've lost a lot of electrolytes.

4. Meal Timing:

The timing of your meals in relation to your workouts can impact your energy levels. A general guideline is to eat a balanced meal 2-3 hours before exercise and a smaller, balanced snack 30 minutes to two hours before.

5. Listen to Your Body:

Pay attention to your body's signals. If you're hungry or fatigued before a workout, eat a small, easily digestible snack to provide energy. During your workout, drink as needed, but avoid overhydration, which can dilute electrolyte levels.

6. Individual Needs:

Nutrition and hydration are highly individual. Your specific needs depend on factors such as your body size, exercise intensity, duration, and personal preferences. Consider consulting with a registered dietitian or nutritionist for personalized guidance.

Optimal nutrition and hydration are fundamental to achieving your fitness goals and maintaining your overall health. By fueling your body with the right nutrients and staying properly hydrated, you can enjoy more effective workouts, quicker recovery, and a healthier, more energized lifestyle

5.1 Fueling Your Body for Workouts

Proper nutrition is the foundation of a successful workout routine. The food you eat provides the energy and nutrients your body needs to perform at its best during exercise, recover afterward, and achieve your fitness goals. Here's how to fuel your body for workouts effectively:

1. Balanced Meals:

Ensure that your daily meals are well-balanced, containing a mix of macronutrients (carbohydrates, proteins, and fats) and micronutrients (vitamins and minerals). This provides a steady source of energy and supports overall health.

2. Pre-WorkoutNutrition:

Fueling your body before exercise is essential for optimal performance. Here's what to consider:

Carbohydrates: Complex carbohydrates like whole grains, fruits, and vegetables are excellent choices. They provide a steady source of energy for your muscles. Consume these foods 1-2 hours before your workout.

Protein: A small amount of lean protein can help with muscle maintenance and growth. Consider including sources like lean meats, yogurt, or legumes in your pre-workout meal or snack.

Hydration: Start your workout well-hydrated. Drink water throughout the day and consider consuming a small amount of water or a sports drink 15-30 minutes before exercising to prevent dehydration.

3. During Exercise Hydration:

Staying properly hydrated during exercise is crucial. Water is usually sufficient for moderate-intensity workouts. If your exercise is intense or prolonged, consider a sports drink to replenish lost electrolytes.

4. Post-Workout Nutrition:

After your workout, your body needs nutrients for recovery and muscle repair. Consider these post-workout nutrition guidelines:

Protein: Consume a source of protein within 30 minutes to two hours after exercise to support muscle recovery. Options include lean meats, poultry, fish, eggs, or plant-based protein sources like tofu or legumes.

Carbohydrates: Replenish glycogen stores by consuming carbohydrates, especially if your workout was intense and prolonged. Whole grains, fruits, and vegetables are excellent choices.

Hydration: Rehydrate by drinking water after your workout to replace any fluids lost during exercise.

5. Meal Timing:

The timing of your meals in relation to your workouts can affect your energy levels. A general guideline is to eat a balanced meal 2-3 hours before exercise and a smaller, balanced snack 30 minutes to two hours before.

6. Listen to Your Body:

Pay attention to your body's signals. If you're hungry or fatigued before a workout, eat a small, easily digestible snack to provide energy. During your workout, drink as needed but avoid overhydration, which can dilute electrolyte levels.

7. Individual Needs:

Nutrition is highly individual. Your specific needs depend on factors like your body size, exercise intensity, and personal preferences. Consulting with a registered dietitian or nutritionist can provide personalized guidance.

Optimal nutrition is crucial to achieving your fitness goals and maintaining overall health. By fueling your body with the right nutrients and staying hydrated, you can enjoy more effective workouts, quicker recovery, and a healthier, more energized lifestyle

5.2 Staying Hydrated for Optimal Performance

Hydration is a fundamental aspect of any successful workout routine. Proper fluid intake is crucial for maintaining energy, focus, and overall physical performance. Whether you're engaged in cardio, strength training, or flexibility exercises, here's why staying hydrated is essential and how to do it effectively:

Importance of Hydration:

Maintaining Energy Levels: Dehydration can lead to a decrease in energy, causing fatigue and reduced endurance during your workouts. Proper hydration ensures that your body has the energy it needs to perform optimally.

Temperature Regulation: Sweating is your body's natural cooling mechanism during exercise. When you're dehydrated, your body struggles to regulate temperature, increasing the risk of overheating and heat-related issues.

Cognitive Function: Dehydration can impair cognitive function, leading to reduced focus and coordination. This can be dangerous, especially during complex exercises or when using gym equipment.

Muscle Function: Water is essential for proper muscle function. Dehydration can lead to muscle cramps and reduced muscle strength, which hampers performance.

Effective Hydration Strategies:

Pre-Hydrate: Start your workout well-hydrated. Drink water throughout the day, especially if you're planning a workout. Aim to consume about 16-20 ounces of water 2-3 hours before your exercise session.

During Exercise Hydration: Depending on the type, intensity, and duration of your workout, you'll have different hydration needs:

For most moderate-intensity workouts, plain water is sufficient. Take small sips regularly during your exercise session.

If you're engaged in prolonged, intense exercise, or you're sweating heavily, consider a sports drink that contains electrolytes like sodium and potassium to replenish lost minerals.

Listen to Your Body: Pay attention to your body's signals. Thirst is a reliable indicator that it's time to drink, but it's better to stay ahead of thirst by taking regular sips of water during your workout.

Rehydrate Post-Workout: After your workout, continue to drink water to replace fluids lost during exercise. The goal is to return to a state of proper hydration. Weigh yourself before and after your workout to estimate how much fluid you've lost, and aim to drink 16-20 ounces of water for every pound lost.

Individualized Approach: Hydration needs vary from person to person. Factors such as body size, workout intensity, temperature, and humidity can all impact your fluid requirements. Consider experimenting to find the hydration strategy that works best for you.

Balanced Diet: In addition to water and sports drinks, remember that you get hydration from various sources in your diet, such as fruits and vegetables, which have a high water content.

Proper hydration is a cornerstone of an effective workout routine. By staying adequately hydrated, you can maintain your energy levels, focus, and physical performance, helping you make the most out of your exercise sessions while minimizing the risk of dehydration-related issues

Chapter 6

Rest and Recovery

Rest and recovery are often underestimated aspects of a successful workout routine. While exercise is crucial for improving fitness, it's during periods of rest and recovery that your body repairs and strengthens, making progress possible. Here's why rest and recovery areessential and how to incorporate them into your fitness plan:

Importance of Rest and Recovery:

Muscle Repair and Growth: When you exercise, you create micro-tears in your muscle fibers. During rest, your body repairs and rebuilds these fibers, making your muscles stronger and more resilient.

Prevention of Overtraining: Excessive exercise without adequate rest can lead to overtraining, characterized by fatigue, decreased performance, and a higher risk of injury. Proper rest helps prevent overtraining and burnout.

Energy Restoration: Rest and sleep allow your body to replenish energy stores, such as glycogen, which is essential for endurance during workouts.

Injury Prevention: Giving your body time to recover helps prevent injuries, as it allows your muscles and joints to heal and reduces the risk of strain and overuse injuries.

Ways to Incorporate Rest and Recovery:

Active Recovery: Active recovery involves low-intensity exercises like walking, cycling, or gentle swimming. Engaging in these activities on rest days can help improve circulation, reduce muscle soreness, and aid recovery.

Sleep: Quality sleep is one of the most critical components of recovery. Aim for 7-9 hours of uninterrupted sleep each night to support muscle repair, hormone balance, and overall well-being.

Nutrition: Proper nutrition plays a vital role in recovery. After a workout, consume a balanced meal or snack that includes protein and carbohydrates to replenish energy and promote muscle repair.

Hydration: Staying well-hydrated supports recovery by helping transport nutrients to muscles and aiding in the removal of waste products.

Stretching and Mobility Work: Incorporating regular stretching and mobility exercises can enhance flexibility and reduce muscle tension, improving overall recovery.

Rest Days: Schedule rest days into your workout plan. These are days when you avoid intense exercise and allow your body to recover. The frequency of rest days may vary, but one to two per week is a common recommendation.

Listening to Your Body: Pay attention to how your body feels. If you're excessively fatigued or experiencing pain, it's a sign that you may need more rest. Don't push through discomfort; instead, allow your body to recover.

Periodization: Incorporate periods of lower-intensity training into your workout plan to give your body a break from high-intensity sessions. This can help prevent overtraining and allow for more extended periods of rest and recovery.

Remember that rest and recovery are not signs of weakness but essential components of a sustainable and effective fitness regimen. By allowing your body the time it needs to recover, you can make better progress, reduce the risk of injury, and enjoy a healthier, more balanced approach to exercise.

6.1 Understanding the Importance of Rest

Rest is a fundamental aspect of life, and its significance extends beyond the context of sleep. It plays a critical role in various aspects of our physical, mental, and emotional well-being. Here's a deeper understanding of the importance of rest:

1. Physical Recovery:

Rest is crucial for the body's physical recovery. During sleep and periods of inactivity, the body undergoes various repair and maintenance processes. This includes the repair and growth of muscle tissues, the release of growth hormones, and the removal of waste products that accumulate during the day. Rest allows your body to heal and rejuvenate, supporting overall physical health and performance.

2. Mental Rejuvenation:

Rest is essential for mental well-being. It provides the brain with the downtime needed to process information, consolidate memories, and recharge cognitive functions. Lack of rest can lead to cognitive deficits, reduced concentration, and an increased risk of mental health issues such as stress, anxiety, and depression.

3. Emotional Balance:

Emotional well-being is closely linked to rest. When you're well-rested, you're better equipped to manage your emotions and cope with stress. Conversely, sleep deprivation and chronic fatigue can lead to mood disturbances and emotional instability.

4. Creativity and Problem Solving:

Rest allows your brain to engage in creative thinking and problem-solving. During moments of rest, your brain can make connections and generate insights that are difficult to achieve in a fatigued state.

5. Immune Function:

Adequate rest is essential for a robust immune system. When you sleep, your body produces immune cells and proteins that help protect against illness and infection. Consistent sleep deprivation can weaken the immune response, making you more susceptible to illnesses.

6. Long-Term Health:

Chronic sleep deprivation and a lack of rest have been linked to various health issues, including cardiovascular disease, obesity, diabetes, and a shortened lifespan. Rest is a cornerstone of long-term health and well-being.

7. Physical Performance:

In the context of exercise and physical performance, rest days are essential. They allow your muscles and joints to recover, reduce the risk of overuse injuries, and promote improved fitness progress.

8. Productivity and Efficiency:

Contrary to the belief that working longer hours leads to increased productivity, rest is essential for efficiency. Adequate rest can lead to better focus, productivity, and job performance.

9. Social and Relationship Well-Being:

Rest also plays a role in maintaining healthy social relationships. When you're well-rested, you're more patient, empathetic, and able to engage positively with others.

In summary, rest is a multifaceted concept with profound implications for physical, mental, emotional, and social well-being. It is not merely a break from activity but a critical component of a healthy and balanced life. Recognizing and prioritizing the importance of rest is essential for maintaining overall health and quality of life

6.2 Recovery Techniques for Effective Workouts

Effective workouts go hand in hand with proper recovery. Ensuring your body can repair, rebuild, and rejuvenate after exercise is essential for achieving fitness goals and preventing injuries. Here are some recovery techniques to help you make the most of your workouts:

1. Sleep:

Quality sleep is the cornerstone of recovery. During sleep, your body engages in critical repair and maintenance processes, including muscle recovery and the release of growth hormones. Aim for 7-9 hours of uninterrupted sleep each night.

2. Hydration:

Proper hydration supports recovery by helping transport nutrients to muscles and aiding in the removal of waste products. Drink water regularly throughout the day and post-workout.

3. Nutrition:

Consuming a balanced meal or snack that includes protein and carbohydrates within 30 minutes to two hours after exercise is vital for muscle recovery. Protein provides amino acids for repair, while carbohydrates replenish energy stores.

4. Active Recovery:

On rest days, engage in low-intensity activities like walking, cycling, or gentle swimming. Active recovery improves circulation, reduces muscle soreness, and enhances recovery.

5. Stretching and Mobility Work:

Regular stretching and mobility exercises improve flexibility, reduce muscle tension, and contribute to overall recovery. Incorporate both dynamic and static stretching into your routine.

6. Foam Rolling and Self-Massage:

Foam rolling can help release muscle knots and improve blood flow to sore areas. Spend time rolling different muscle groups post-workout to reduce muscle tightness.

7. Ice Baths and Contrast Baths:

Alternating between hot and cold baths or showers (contrast baths) can reduce muscle soreness and inflammation. Cold baths can also be effective for specific injuries or sore spots.

8. Compression Garments:

Wearing compression garments like sleeves, socks, or shirts can help improve blood flow and reduce muscle swelling, which can enhance recovery.

9. Epsom Salt Baths:

Epsom salt baths can soothe sore muscles and reduce muscle cramps. The magnesium in Epsom salts can be absorbed through the skin, providing additional benefits.

10. Rest Days:

Incorporate rest days into your workout plan. These are days when you avoid intense exercise, allowing your body to recover. The frequency of rest days may vary but typically includes one to two per week.

11. Listening to Your Body:

Pay attention to how your body feels. If you're excessively fatigued or experiencing pain, it's a sign that you may need more rest. Don't push through discomfort; instead, allow your body to recover.

12. Periodization:

Periodization involves incorporating periods of lower-intensity training into your workout plan to give your body a break from high-intensity sessions. This can help prevent overtraining and allow for more extended periods of rest and recovery.

Remember that recovery is an individual process. Listen to your body and adjust your recovery techniques as needed. By prioritizing recovery, you can maximize the benefits of your workouts, reduce the risk of injuries, and achieve your fitness goals more effectively

Chapter 7

Staying Motivated

Maintaining motivation is often one of the biggest challenges when it comes to sticking to a workout routine. Whether you're just starting or have been exercising for a while, motivation can ebb and flow. Here are some strategies to help you stay motivated and committed to your fitness goals:

1. Set Clear and Achievable Goals:

Define specific, realistic, and time-bound goals. Whether it's running a certain distance, lifting a particular weight, or losing a specific amount of weight, having clear objectives gives you something to work toward.

2. Create a Workout Schedule:

Plan your workouts in advance and schedule them like appointments. This commitment can help you stick to your routine and avoid procrastination.

3. Find What You Enjoy:

Engage in activities you genuinely enjoy. Whether it's dancing, hiking, swimming, or practicing yoga, doing things you love makes it easier to stay motivated.

4. Vary Your Routine:

Monotony can lead to boredom and reduced motivation. Change up your workouts by incorporating different exercises, classes, or outdoor activities to keep things fresh and exciting.

5. Exercise with a Buddy:

Working out with a friend or joining a group fitness class can provide accountability and make exercise more enjoyable. The social aspect can boost motivation.

6. Use Technology:

Fitness apps and wearables can track your progress, provide motivation, and offer a sense of achievement. Set challenges and compete with yourself to reach new milestones.

7. Reward Yourself:

Treat yourself when you achieve a milestone. Rewards can serve as positive reinforcement for your efforts and keep you motivated.

8. Visualize Success:

Imagine the benefits of achieving your fitness goals. Visualizing yourself healthier, stronger, or more energetic can be a powerful motivator.

9. Track Your Progress:

Keep a workout journal to monitor your progress. Seeing improvements over time, whether it's lifting more weight, running faster, or losing weight, can be highly motivating.

10. Embrace the "No Excuses" Mindset:

Understand that there will always be obstacles and excuses. Recognize them, but don't let them derail your motivation. Commit to your goals, even on days when you're not feeling 100%.

11. Find Inspiration:

Follow fitness influencers, read books, or watch documentaries that inspire you. Learning about others' journeys can motivate you to continue your own.

12. Focus on the Journey, Not Just the Destination:

Instead of fixating on end results, focus on the daily enjoyment, sense of accomplishment, and positive feelings you get from exercise.

13. Seek Professional Guidance:

Consider working with a personal trainer, coach, or nutritionist. They can provide expert guidance, personalized plans, and accountability.

14. Be Patient and Kind to Yourself:

Acknowledge that progress takes time and that there will be setbacks. Be patient and avoid being overly critical if you miss a workout or indulge in an occasional treat.

15. Adapt and Evolve:

Be open to changing your workout routine as your interests and goals evolve. This can prevent staleness and reignite your motivation.

Remember that motivation can fluctuate, but with these strategies and a consistent commitment to your goals, you can maintain the drive to stick to your workout routine and achieve lasting fitness success

7.1 Finding Motivation to Stick to Your Routine

Staying motivated to adhere to your fitness routine can be a challenging endeavor, but there are numerous strategies to help you maintain your commitment and achieve your goals. Here are some tips for finding and sustaining motivation:

1. Define Your "Why":

Understanding the reasons behind your desire to exercise is a powerful motivator. Whether it's improved health, increased energy, weight loss, or a specific fitness goal, knowing your "why" can help you stay focused.

2. Set Clear and Achievable Goals:

Establish specific, measurable, and realistic fitness goals. Break down your long-term goals into smaller, more achievable milestones. Tracking your progress and celebrating each accomplishment can be motivating.

3. Create a Structured Plan:

Develop a well-structured workout plan. Having a set schedule and knowing exactly what you're going to do during each session can reduce uncertainty and make it easier to stick to your routine.

4. Mix It Up:

Variety can keep your workouts interesting. Incorporate different types of exercises, classes, or outdoor activities to prevent boredom and maintain motivation.

5. Find Enjoyment:

Discover physical activities you genuinely enjoy. If you like what you're doing, you're more likely to stick with it. Try various sports, dance, or fitness classes until you find what resonates with you.

6. Make It Social:

Working out with a friend or joining group fitness classes can make exercise more enjoyable. The social aspect can provide motivation, support, and accountability.

7. Use Technology:

Fitness apps, trackers, and wearables can monitor
your progress, set challenges, and provide motivation through data and feedback.

8. Reward Yourself:

Set up a reward system for reaching milestones. Treat yourself to something you enjoy when you achieve a goal. This provides positive reinforcement for your efforts.

9. Visualize Success:

Spend time visualizing the benefits of achieving your fitness goals. See yourself healthier, stronger, and happier. Visualizations can be a powerful motivator.

10. Track Your Progress:

Maintain a workout journal to record your achievements and setbacks. Seeing improvements over time can boost motivation and confidence.

11. Overcome Excuses:

Recognize that there will always be obstacles and excuses. Accept them as part of the journey but don't let them become roadblocks. Commit to your goals, even on challenging days.

12. Focus on Health and Well-Being:

Shift your perspective from just the aesthetics of exercise to the overall health and well-being it provides. Feeling healthier, more energetic, and less stressed can be strong motivators.

13. Learn from Others:

Follow fitness influencers, read books, or watch documentaries about inspiring fitness journeys. Learning about the experiences of others can motivate you to continue your own.

14. Embrace the "No Excuses" Mindset:

Understand that no excuse is insurmountable. Commit to your goals and adopt a mindset that refuses to accept excuses.

15. Seek Professional Guidance:

Consider working with a personal trainer, coach, or nutritionist. They can provide expert guidance, personalized plans, and accountability.

16. Be Patient and Kind to Yourself:

Acknowledge that progress takes time and that setbacks are part of the journey. Be patient and practice self-compassion.

17. Adapt and Evolve:

Be open to changing your workout routine as your interests and goals evolve. This can prevent staleness and maintain your motivation.

Remember that motivation may fluctuate, but with a combination of these strategies and a steadfast commitment to your goals, you can maintain your motivation and achieve long-lasting success in your fitness routine

7.2 Overcoming Challenges and Plateaus

In your fitness journey, you're likely to encounter challenges and plateaus that can test your motivation and progress. Here's how to overcome them and keep moving forward:

1. Identify the Challenge:

The first step in overcoming any obstacle is to clearly identify it. Is it a lack of motivation, a specific fitness plateau, an injury, or a scheduling issue? Understanding the challenge is crucial for finding the right solution.

2. Revise Your Goals:

Reevaluate your fitness goals. Are they still relevant, or do you need to adjust them? Setting new goals or modifying existing ones can reignite your motivation and provide a fresh sense of purpose.

3. Seek Support:

Don't be afraid to ask for help. Join a fitness group, work with a personal trainer, or consult a coach or physical therapist for guidance and support. Having someone in your corner can make a significant difference.

4. Change Your Routine:

Variation can break plateaus. Alter your workout routine by trying new exercises, different intensities, or varying the order of your workouts. This challenges your body and can lead to progress.

5. Nutrition and Hydration:

Review your diet and hydration. Proper nutrition and hydration are vital for your performance. Ensure you're fueling your body with the right nutrients and staying adequately hydrated.

6. Rest and Recovery:

Consider your rest and recovery. Overtraining can lead to plateaus and injuries. Allow your body time to recover, and ensure you're getting enough sleep.

7. Set Short-Term Goals:

In additionto long-term goals, set short-term goals to track your progress. These can help you stay motivated and focused on achievable milestones.

8. Embrace Cross-Training:

Incorporate cross-training into your routine. Activities like swimming, cycling, or yoga can help target different muscle groups and offer a break from the monotony of your primary workout.

9. Mindset and Visualization:

Cultivate a positive mindset. Visualization techniques can help you see and believe in your success. Envision yourself breaking through plateaus and achieving your goals.

10. Stay Consistent:

Consistency is key. Plateaus can be a result of inconsistency in your workout routine. Make exercise a regular part of your life to maintain progress.

11. Keep a Journal:

Maintain a workout journal to track your exercises, nutrition, and progress. This can provide insights into what's working and what might need adjustment.

12. Celebrate Small Wins:

Don't wait for major accomplishments to celebrate. Recognize and reward yourself for small achievements and milestones along the way.

13. Be Patient:

Plateaus are a natural part of the fitness journey. Be patient and remember that progress may be slow at times. Stay committed to your goals.

14. Stay Positive:

Maintain a positive attitude. A negative outlook can hinder progress. Stay focused on the benefits and improvements you've already experienced.

15. Remember Your "Why":

Revisit your initial motivation and the reasons you started your fitness journey. Reconnecting with your "why" can reignite your determination.

16. Consult a Professional:

If you're dealing with an injury or specific fitness challenge, seek guidance from a healthcare professional or fitness expert. They can provide personalized solutions.

17. Don't Give Up:

Above all, don't give up. Plateaus and challenges are part of the process. Keep moving forward, stay resilient, and remember that consistency and determination can lead to breakthroughs.

Overcoming challenges and plateaus is a natural part of your fitness journey. By applying these strategies and staying committed to your goals, you can continue to make progress and achieve the results you desire

Chapter 8

Tracking Progress

Tracking your progress is a fundamental aspect of a successful fitness journey. It allows you to monitor your development, stay motivated, and make informed decisions about your workout routine and nutrition. Here's why tracking progress is essential and how to do it effectively:

Why Track Your Progress:

Motivation: Seeing tangible evidence of your progress can boost your motivation and reinforce your commitment to your fitness goals.

Accountability: Tracking keeps you accountable. It reminds you of your goals and encourages consistency in your workouts and nutrition.

Feedback: Regular progress monitoring provides valuable feedback on what is working and what might need adjustment in your routine.
Goal Assessment: It helps you assess whether you're on track to meet your fitness goals. If not, it allows you to make necessary changes.

Recognizing Plateaus: Plateaus are common in fitness. Tracking can help you identify when progress slows down, allowing you to adapt and overcome plateaus.

Improves Efficiency: By knowing what works best for you, you can optimize your fitness routine, making it more efficient and tailored to your needs.

How to Track Your Progress:

Fitness Journal: Keep a detailed journal of your workouts, including exercises, sets, reps, and weights used. Write down your feelings, energy levels, and any challenges you faced during the workout.

Measurements: Regularly measure key metrics like body weight, body fat percentage, waist circumference, and other relevant body measurements.

Photographs: Take progress photos from various angles to visually track changes in your physique over time.

Performance Metrics: Track your performance improvements, such as lifting heavier weights, running faster times, or completing more reps. Use apps, workout logs, or spreadsheets to record these metrics.

Nutrition: Maintain a food diary to record what you eat and drink. Tracking your nutrition can help you identify dietary patterns and make healthier choices.

Health and Well-Being: Note changes in your overall health and well-being, such as increased energy, better sleep, or reduced stress levels.

Body Composition Scans: Consider using body composition scans, like DEXA or bioelectrical impedance analysis, to assess muscle mass and body fat percentage more accurately.

Fitness Apps and Wearables: Use fitness apps and wearable devices to monitor your steps, heart rate, and other relevant data. Many of these apps provide a comprehensive overview of your fitness journey.

Regular Assessments: Schedule regular assessments with a fitness professional, like a personal trainer or dietitian, to evaluate your progress and get expert feedback.

Goal Setting: Set specific, measurable goals and timelines for achieving them. Regularly review your progress in relation to these goals.

Reflect and Adapt: Periodically analyze your progress data. If you notice a lack of progress or setbacks, adapt your routine or seek professional guidance.

Stay Consistent: The key to effective progress tracking is consistency. Record data regularly, so you have a comprehensive history to review.

Remember that progress in your fitness journey can be gradual and nonlinear. Plateaus and setbacks are normal. The key is to stay committed, stay patient, and use progress tracking as a valuable tool to help you make informed decisions and reach your fitness goals

8.1 Monitoring Your Progress and Adjusting Your Routine

Monitoring your progress and making necessary adjustments to your fitness routine is a vital part of achieving your health and fitness goals. Here's how to effectively track your progress and adapt your routine for continued success:

1. Establish Baseline Data:

Start by gathering baseline data to understand your current fitness level. This might include measurements, body composition, fitness assessments, and a record of your current exercise and eating habits.

2. Set Clear Goals:

Define specific, measurable, achievable, relevant, and time-bound (SMART) goals. Your goals should be the guiding force behind your fitness journey.

3. Choose Progress Tracking Methods:

Select the methods for tracking your progress. This might include keeping a fitness journal, using workout logs, measuring body weight and body composition, monitoring performance improvements, or using fitness apps and wearables.

4. RegularAssessment:

Schedule regular assessments. This can be weekly, monthly, or based on the nature of your goals. Assessments will help you see patterns and trends in your progress.

5. Analyze Your Data:

Review your progress data periodically. Look for trends, areas where you're excelling, and areas that need improvement. Consider how your progress aligns with your goals.

6. Celebrate Achievements:

Recognize and celebrate your achievements and milestones. Positive reinforcement can boost your motivation and sense of accomplishment.

7. Adjust Your Routine:

If you're not progressing as desired or have hit a plateau, it's time to adjust your routine. Here's how:

Change Exercises: Introduce new exercises or variations to target different muscle groups and prevent overuse injuries.

Modify Intensity: Adjust the intensity of your workouts. Increase resistance, change your cardio intervals, or explore high-intensity interval training (HIIT).

Tweak Frequency: Alter the frequency of your workouts. You might need more or less depending on your goals and progress.

Adjust Duration: Change the duration of your workouts. Longer workouts may be necessary for certain goals, while shorter, intense sessions might be more effective for others.

Diet and Nutrition: Reevaluate your nutrition. Are you consuming enough calories and nutrients to support your goals? Adjust your diet as necessary.

Rest and Recovery: Ensure you're getting enough rest and recovery. Overtraining can lead to plateaus and injuries.

Consult a Professional: Seek advice from a fitness trainer, dietitian, or healthcare professional. They can provide expert guidance on making the right adjustments.

8. Stay Patient:

Remember that progress isn't always linear. Plateaus and setbacks are common in any fitness journey. Be patient and persistent.

9. Periodically Reassess:

Reassess your goals and your progress tracking methods. As you evolve, your goals and the way you track progress may need to evolve as well.

10. Stay Consistent:

Consistency is key. Continue to track your progress and make adjustments as necessary to maintain your fitness gains and work toward your goals.

By actively monitoring your progress and making informed adjustments, you can adapt your fitness routine to keep moving in the right direction. Whether your goals are related to strength, endurance, weight loss, or overall health, this process ensures that you're on the path to success

8.2 Celebrating Achievements Along the Way

Celebrating your achievements, no matter how small, is a powerful way to maintain motivation and a positive mindset on your fitness journey. Here's why celebrating achievements is crucial and how to do it effectively:

The Importance of Celebration:

Motivation: Celebrating achievements provides a sense of accomplishment and reinforces your motivation to continue working toward your goals.

Positive Reinforcement: Recognizing your progress with celebration is a form of positive reinforcement, which encourages you to repeat the behaviors that led to your achievements.

Mental and Emotional Well-Being: Celebrating milestones boosts your mental and emotional well-being. It enhances your self-esteem and confidence, reducing stress and anxiety.

Long-Term Commitment: Consistent recognitionachievements helps maintain your long-term commitment to your fitness goals, as it keeps your enthusiasm and determination high.

Effective Ways to Celebrate Achievements:

Acknowledge Small Wins: Don't wait for major accomplishments to celebrate. Recognize and applaud even the smallest victories, like completing a challenging workout, increasing the weight you lift, or sticking to your nutrition plan for a week.

Set Milestone Rewards: Create a system of rewards for reaching specific milestones or goals. It could be a treat, a fun activity, or anything that brings you joy.

Share Your Success: Share your achievements with friends, family, or a support group. Their encouragement and acknowledgment can make your successes even more meaningful.

Visualize Your Progress: Create a vision board or journal to visually track your achievements. Document your journey with photos and notes to remind yourself of how far you've come.

Reflect on Your Journey: Take time to reflect on your achievements, reminding yourself of the hard work and dedication that got you there. Journal about your journey and how it has positively impacted your life.

Upgrade Your Gear: As a reward for your achievements, consider upgrading your fitness gear, whether it's a new workout outfit, running shoes, or fitness equipment.

Give Back: Celebrate your accomplishments by giving back. Participate in a charity run, volunteer at a fitness event, or help a friend get started on their fitness journey.

Plan a Fitness Adventure: Celebrate with a fitness adventure or event. Sign up for a race, participate in a challenging hike, or take a weekend trip centered around physical activities.

Enjoy a Relaxing Treat: Treat yourself to a day of relaxation, whether it's a spa day, a massage, or a wellness retreat. Recovery is part of the fitness journey, and relaxation can be a form of celebration.

Public Commitment: Share your goals and achievements on social media or in a blog. The public commitment can provide an added layer of motivation and accountability.

Create Your Traditions: Develop your unique traditions or rituals for celebrating achievements. These personal rituals can become meaningful markers of your progress.

Surround Yourself with Positivity: Spend time with positive people who support and celebrate your achievements. Their enthusiasm can be contagious.

Celebrating achievements is a fundamental part of enjoying your fitness journey. It keeps you engaged, motivated, and excited about the process. Recognizing your progress, no matter how small, is a testament to your dedication and hard work. It's a reminder of your potential for continued success and growth in your fitness pursuits

Chapter 9

Incorporating Sustainable Practices

In addition to improving your physical health and well-being, it's important to consider the environmental and ethical impact of your fitness journey. Here are ways to incorporate sustainable practices into your fitness routine:

1. Sustainable Gear:

Invest in eco-friendly workout gear made from sustainable materials. Look for brands that prioritize eco-conscious manufacturing processes and materials like organic cotton, recycled polyester, and sustainable fabrics.

2. Eco-Friendly Transportation:

Choose sustainable transportation options to get to your workouts. Walk, bike, carpool, or use public transportation to reduce your carbon footprint when traveling to the gym or your favorite outdoor exercise spot.

3. Choose Eco-Friendly Fitness Facilities:

If possible, select fitness facilities that have adopted sustainable practices. These include gyms that use energy-efficient equipment, recycle, and minimize water waste.

4. Outdoor Workouts:

Opt for outdoor workouts when weather and location permit. Parks and natural settings provide a beautiful backdrop for your fitness routine and have a lower environmental impact than indoor facilities.

5. Sustainable Nutrition:

Support sustainable agriculture by choosing locally sourced and organic foods. Reducing the carbon footprint of your meals can complement your fitness efforts by promoting a healthier planet

6. Reusable Water Bottles and Containers:

Minimize single-use plastic waste by using reusable water bottles and containers for your pre- and post-workout snacks. This practice reduces plastic pollution and saves money in the long run.

7. Recycle and Compost:

Properly dispose of your waste. Recycle items like protein bar wrappers and packaging materials. If available, compost organic waste from your nutrition and meal prep.

8. Sustainable Hydration:

Choose a reusable and eco-friendly water bottle, and opt for water sources that reduce single-use plastic waste. You can also explore water filtration options to reduce reliance on bottled water.

9. Energy-Efficient Workouts:

Consider energy-efficient workout routines. Utilize bodyweight exercises and minimal equipment to reduce the need for energy-consuming machines or devices.

10. Support Sustainable Brands:

Choose fitness and sportswear brands that prioritize sustainability, such as companies committed to reducing their carbon footprint, using sustainable materials, and ethical labor practices.

11. Minimize Gym Waste:

If you work out at a gym, be mindful of your waste production. Use a reusable gym towel and bring your own eco-friendly, refillable toiletries.

12. Choose Eco-Friendly Fitness Classes:

Select fitness classes or programs that integrate environmental consciousness into their routines. These might include outdoor yoga sessions, eco-friendly boot camps, or group hikes.

13. Reduce Water Waste:

Conserve water during your workouts and post-workout routines. Use a sweat towel rather than taking excessive showers to reduce water usage.

14. Donate or Resell Unused Gear:

Rather than discarding old workout equipment and clothing, donate it to local organizations or resell it. This extends the lifespan of these items and reduces waste.

15. Conscious Nutrition Choices:

Consider adopting a more plant-based or sustainable diet. Reducing meat consumption, particularly from industrial farming, can have a significant positive impact on the environment.

Incorporating sustainable practices into your fitness routine not only benefits the planet but also enhances your holistic well-being. By making eco-conscious choices, you align your fitness journey with broader efforts to create a healthier, more sustainable world for yourself and future generations

9.1 Environmentally Friendly Workout Tips

Taking care of the environment doesn't have to be at odds with your fitness routine. You can adopt environmentally friendly workout practices that reduce your carbon footprint and minimize your impact on the planet. Here are some tips:

1. Choose Outdoor Workouts:

Opt for outdoor workouts whenever possible. Exercising in natural settings like parks, forests, and beaches not only reduces the need for electricity but also allows you to connect with nature.

2. Sustainable Activewear:

Invest in activewear made from sustainable and eco-friendly materials. Look for brands that use recycled materials, organic fabrics, and ethical manufacturing processes.

3. Eco-Friendly Transport:

Walk, bike, or use public transportation to get to your workouts. Reduce emissions by avoiding unnecessary car trips to the gym or fitness classes.

4. Reusable Water Bottles:

Ditch single-use plastic water bottles and invest in a reusable one. Fill it with tap water or use a water filtration system to reduce plastic waste.

5. Recycle Workout Gear:

Recycle old workout gear and equipment responsibly. Many fitness centers and organizations collect and recycle used fitness equipment. Look for local options to donate or recycle your old gear.

6. Sustainable Nutrition:

Embrace a sustainable diet by choosing locally sourced, seasonal, and organic foods. Reducing your carbon footprint through nutrition complements your fitness efforts.

7. Energy-Efficient Workouts:

Opt for energy-efficient workout routines. Bodyweight exercises, minimal equipment workouts, and high-intensity interval training (HIIT) are effective ways to reduce your reliance on energy-consuming machines.

8. Minimize Shower Time:

After your workout, consider taking shorter, cooler showers to save water and energy. Use a sweat towel to freshen up instead of a full shower when it's feasible.

9. Eco-Friendly Workouts at Home:

If you prefer home workouts, invest in energy-efficient workout equipment and use energy-efficient light bulbs and appliances in your workout space.

10. Power from Renewable Sources:

If you use electronic devices during your workouts, consider powering them with electricity from renewable sources. Opt for solar-powered chargers or choose an energy provider that uses renewable energy.

11. Public Transportation to Fitness Classes:

When attending fitness classes or group workouts, choose public transportation, carpool, or bike to the location to reduce emissions from individual vehicles.

12. Gym Towels:

If you go to a gym, use reusable towels instead of disposable ones. Many gyms offer cloth towels that can be used during your workout and then laundered for the next user.

13. Resale or Donation:

If you're upgrading your fitness equipment or apparel, consider reselling or donating your old items. This extends their lifecycle and reduces waste.

14. Reduce and Reuse:

Embrace the reduce and reuse principles in your fitness journey. Use a refillable water bottle, reduce plastic waste, and find ways to repurpose items.

15. Support Green Gyms:

Seek out gyms and fitness facilities that have adopted sustainable practices, such as energy-efficient equipment and waste reduction programs.

16. Organized Group Eco Workouts:

Join or organize group eco workouts like beach cleanups, nature hikes, or eco-friendly races that promote environmental awareness.

By incorporating these environmentally friendly workout tips into your fitness routine, you can contribute to a more sustainable and eco-conscious approach to health and well-being. It's a win-win situation that benefits both your personal fitness goals and the planet

9.2 Mindful Approaches to Exercise for Long-term Commitment

To maintain a long-term commitment to exercise, it's essential to adopt mindful and sustainable practices that make fitness a consistent and enjoyable part of your life. Here are some approaches to help you stay committed to your exercise routine:

1. Set Realistic Goals:

Start with achievable, realistic fitness goals. Setting the bar too high can lead to frustration and burnout. Gradually progress and celebrate small victories along the way.

2. Find Activities You Love:

Choose physical activities you genuinely enjoy. Whether it's dancing, hiking, swimming, or practicing yoga, doing something you love makes it easier to stay committed.

3. Embrace Mindfulness:

Practice mindfulness during your workouts. Pay attention to your body, your movements, and your breathing. This enhances the mind-body connection and can make your workouts more enjoyable.

4. Make Exercise a Habit:

Consistency is key. Establish a routine that incorporates exercise into your daily or weekly schedule, making it a natural part of your life.

5. Set a Workout Schedule:

Plan your workouts in advance and schedule them like appointments. This commitment can help you stick to your routine and avoid procrastination.

6. Vary Your Routine:

Monotony can lead to boredom and reduced commitment. Change up your workouts by incorporating different exercises, classes, or outdoor activities to keep things fresh and exciting.

7. Listen to Your Body:

Pay attention to how your body feels. If you're excessively fatigued or experiencing pain, it's a sign that you may need more rest. Don't push through discomfort; instead, allow your body to recover.

8. Prioritize Quality Over Quantity:

Quality of exercise is more important than quantity. A focused, effective 30-minute workout can be as beneficial as a longer, less focused one.

9. Set Short-Term Goals:

In addition to long-term goals, set short-term goals to track your progress. These can help you stay motivated and focused on achievable milestones.

10. Partner Up:

Exercise with a friend or join a group fitness class. The social aspect can provide accountability and make exercise more enjoyable.

11. Reward Yourself:

Treat yourself when you achieve a milestone. Rewards can serve as positive reinforcement for your efforts and keep you motivated.

12. Practice Patience:

Understand that progress takes time. Be patient with yourself and avoid being overly critical if you miss a workout or indulge in an occasional treat.

13. Focus on the Journey, Not Just the Destination:

Instead of fixating on end results, focus on the daily enjoyment, sense of accomplishment, and positive feelings you get from exercise.

14. Be Open to Change:

Be open to changing your workout routine as your interests and goals evolve. This can prevent staleness and maintain your commitment.

15. Seek Professional Guidance:

Consider working with a personal trainer, coach, or nutritionist. They can provide expert guidance, personalized plans, and accountability.

By adopting mindful approaches to exercise, you can build a long-term commitment to fitness that extends well beyond immediate goals. Exercise becomes a part of your lifestyle, contributing to your overall well-being and happiness

Chapter 10

Additional Resources

In addition to the valuable insights provided in this guide, there are numerous additional resources that can further support and enhance your fitness journey. Here are some resources to consider:

1. Fitness Apps:

MyFitnessPal: A comprehensive fitness and nutrition tracker.
Nike Training Club: Offers a wide range of workout plans and guided workouts.
Strava: Great for tracking and sharing your outdoor workouts.

2. Online Fitness Communities:

Reddit's r/Fitness: A vast community for fitness enthusiasts.
Bodybuilding.com: Forums and articles on a wide range of fitness topics.
Fitbit Community: A place to connect with other Fitbit users and find workout inspiration.

3. Books and Magazines:

"Born to Run" by Christopher McDougall: An inspiring book about running and endurance.

"The New Rules of Lifting" by Lou Schuler and Alwyn Cosgrove: A guide to strength training.

Fitness magazines like Men's Health, Women's Health, and Runner's World offer workout ideas and expert advice.

4. Podcasts:

"The Joe Rogan Experience": Features interviews with fitness experts and athletes.

"The Model Health Show" by Shawn Stevenson: Focuses on health and wellness topics.

"Mind Pump: Raw Fitness Truth": Offers fitness, nutrition, and health insights.

5. YouTube Channels:

FitnessBlender: Provides a wide variety of free workout videos.

Athlean-X: Focuses on strength training and injury prevention.

Yoga with Adriene: Offers yoga routines for all levels.

6. Fitness Professionals:

Consider working with a certified personal trainer, nutritionist, or physical therapist for personalized guidance.

7. Local Fitness Classes:

Check out local gyms, studios, and community centers for group fitness classes like yoga, HIIT, spinning, or dance.

8. Wearable Technology:

Fitness trackers like Fitbit, Garmin, or Apple Watch can help you monitor your activity and progress.
9. Social Media:

Follow fitness influencers and experts on platforms like Instagram and TikTok for workout inspiration and tips.

10. Cooking and Nutrition Resources:

Explore cookbooks and online recipes to support your healthy eating goals. Websites like AllRecipes and Food Network offer a wealth of recipes.

11. Medical Professionals:

Consult with healthcare providers, including doctors, dietitians, and physical therapists, for personalized advice and guidance.
12. Online Courses and Certifications:

If you want to deepen your fitness knowledge, consider taking online courses or obtaining certifications in areas like personal training, nutrition, or yoga instruction.

Remember that your fitness journey is personal, and the resources you choose should align with your specific goals and interests. Whether you're looking to build strength, increase endurance, lose weight, or simply improve your overall health, these additional resources can provide you with the knowledge, support, and motivation needed to achieve success

10.1 Recommended Reading and References

To further your understanding of fitness and health, consider delving into these recommended reading materials and references. These books and sources offer valuable insights and knowledge to support your fitness journey:

1. "Born to Run" by Christopher McDougall:

A captivating exploration of human endurance and the joy of running. This book inspires a deep appreciation for the sport of running.

2. "The New Rules of Lifting" by Lou Schuler and Alwyn Cosgrove:

An informative guide to strength training, offering practical advice for those looking to build muscle, lose weight, and improve overall fitness.

3. "Spark: The Revolutionary New Science of Exercise and the Brain" by John J. Ratey:

This book delves into the profound effects of exercise on brain health, mood, and cognitive function.

4. "Becoming a Supple Leopard" by Dr. Kelly Starrett:

A comprehensive resource on mobility and movement, focusing on techniques to prevent injuries and optimize performance.

5. "The Fitness Mindset" by Brian Keane:

Offers insights into the psychology of fitness, motivation, and the habits that lead to long-term success.

6. "Good Calories, Bad Calories" by Gary Taubes:

A thought-provoking book that challenges common beliefs about nutrition and weight loss, examining the science behind diet and exercise.

7. "Precision Nutrition" by John Berardi:

A comprehensive guide to nutrition and healthy eating, including strategies for achieving your fitness and wellness goals.

8. "The Power of Habit" by Charles Duhigg:

Explores the science of habit formation and how habits influence our fitness routines and overall health.

9. "Thrive" by Brendan Brazier:

A plant-based nutrition guide that provides insights into fueling your body for optimal performance.

10. Scientific Journals and Websites:

Access reputable sources like PubMed, WebMD, and journals like the American College of Sports Medicine's "Medicine & Science in Sports & Exercise" for the latest research and studies on exercise, nutrition, and health.

11. Personalized Resources:

Consult with personal trainers, dietitians, and medical professionals who can offer guidance tailored to your unique needs and goals.

12. Online Fitness Communities and Forums:

Engage with fitness enthusiasts and experts on platforms like Reddit's r/Fitness and Bodybuilding.com forums to ask questions and share experiences.

These resources provide a well-rounded foundation of knowledge to support your fitness journey. Remember that every individual's fitness path is unique, so feel free to explore these references to find the information and strategies that align with your goals and interests

www.ingramcontent.com/pod-product-compliance
Lightning Source LLC
Chambersburg PA
CBHW071608270726

48661CB00019B/1649